The Comprehensive Plant-Based Dinner Cookbook

A Complete Collection of Plant-Based Recipes to Enjoy Your Diet and Boost Your Health

Toby Hancock

Table of contents

Simple Almond Butter Fudge

Preparation Time: 15 minutes Serves: 8

Ingredients:

1/2 cup almond butter 15 drops liquid stevia 2 1/2 tbsp coconut oil

Directions:

Combine together almond butter and coconut oil in a saucepan. Gently warm until melted. Add stevia and stir well. Pour mixture into the candy container and place in refrigerator until set. Serve and enjoy.

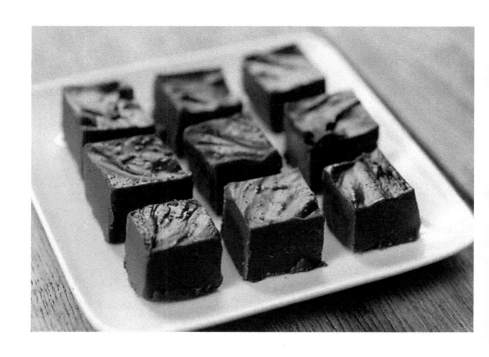

Lemon Mousse

Preparation Time: 10 minutes Serves: 2

Ingredients:

14 oz coconut milk 12 drops liquid stevia 1/2 tsp lemon extract 1/4 tsp turmeric

Directions:

Place coconut milk can in the refrigerator for overnight. Scoop out thick cream into a mixing bowl. Add remaining Ingredients to the bowl and whip using a hand mixer until smooth. Transfer mousse mixture to a zip-lock bag and pipe into small serving glasses. Place in refrigerator. Serve chilled and enjoy.

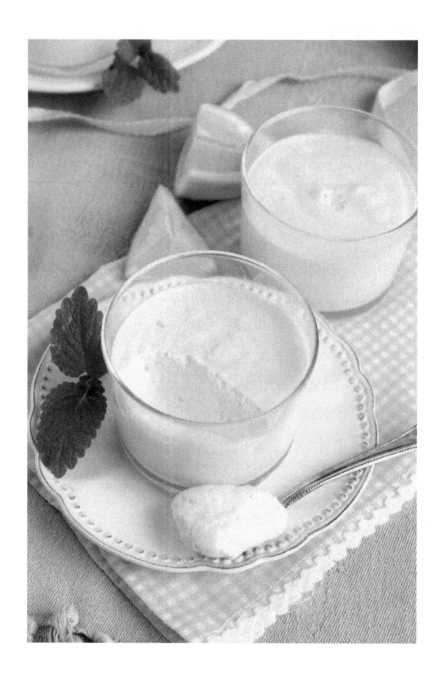

Veggie & Tofu Kebabs

Preparation Time: 15 minutes Cooking Time: 12 minutes Servings: 4

Ingredients:

2 cloves garlic, minced ¼ cup balsamic vinegar ¼ cup olive oil 1 tablespoon Italian seasoning Salt and pepper to taste 1 onion, sliced into quarters 12 medium mushrooms 16 cherry tomatoes 1 zucchini, sliced into rounds 1 cup tofu, cubed 4 cups cauliflower rice

Direction

In a bowl, mix the garlic, vinegar, oil, Italian seasoning, salt and pepper. Toss the vegetable slices and tofu in the mixture. Marinate for 1 hour. Thread into 8 skewers and grill for 12 minutes, turning once or twice. Add cauliflower rice into 4 food containers. Add 2 kebab skewers on top of each container of cauliflower rice. Reheat kebabs in the grill before serving.

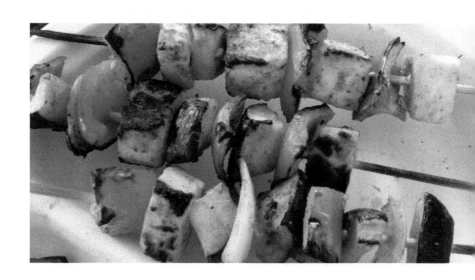

Spicy Snow Pea and Tofu Stir Fry

Preparation Time: 20 minutes Cooking Time: 20 minutes

Servings: 4

Ingredients:

1 cup unsalted natural peanut butter

2 teaspoons brown sugar

2 tablespoons reduced-sodium soy sauce

2 teaspoons hot sauce

3 tablespoons rice vinegar

14 oz. tofu 4 teaspoons oil

1/4 cup onion, sliced

2 tablespoons ginger, grated

3 cloves garlic, minced

1/2 cup broccoli, sliced into florets

1/2 cup carrot, sliced into sticks

2 cups fresh snow peas, trimmed

2 tablespoons water

2 cups brown rice, cooked

4 tablespoons roasted peanuts (unsalted)

Direction In a bowl, mix the peanut butter, sugar, soy sauce, hot sauce and rice vinegar. Blend until smooth and set aside. Drain the tofu and sliced into cubes. Pat dry with paper towel. Add oil to a pan over medium heat. Add the tofu and cook for 2 minutes or until brown on all sides. Transfer the tofu to a plate. Add the onion, ginger and garlic to the pan. Cook for 2 minutes. Add the broccoli and carrot. Cook for 5 minutes. Stir in the snow peas. Pour in the water and cover. Cook for 4 minutes. Add the peanut sauce to the pan along with the tofu. Heat through for 30 seconds. In a food container, add the brown rice and top with the tofu and vegetable stir fry. Top with roasted peanuts.

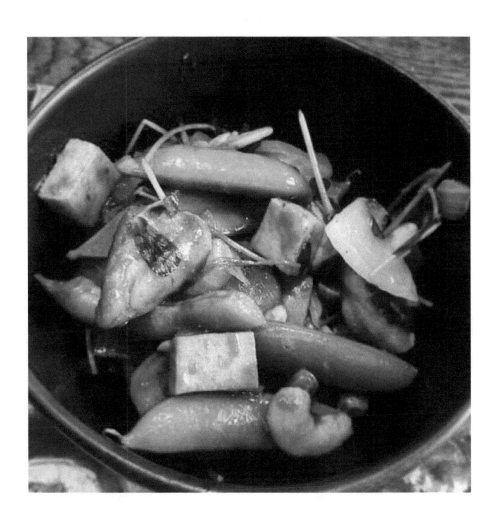

Spinach with Walnuts & Avocado

Preparation Time: 5 minutes Cooking Time: 0 minute
Servings: 1

Ingredients:

3 cups baby spinach ½ cup strawberries, sliced 1 tablespoon white onion, chopped 2 tablespoons vinaigrette ¼ medium avocado, diced 2 tablespoons walnut, toasted

Direction

Put the spinach, strawberries and onion in a glass jar with lid. Drizzle dressing on top. Top with avocado and walnuts. Seal the lid and refrigerate until ready to serve.

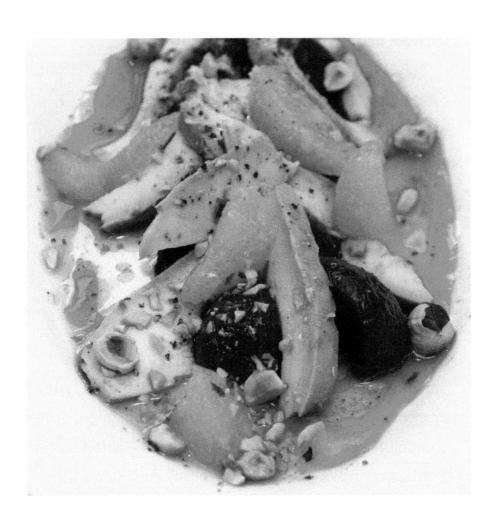

Grilled Broccoli with Chili Garlic Oil

Preparation Time: 15 minutes Cooking Time: 16 minutes

Servings: 4

Ingredients:

3 tablespoons olive oil, divided 2 tablespoons vegetable broth (unsalted) 2 cloves garlic, sliced thinly 1 chili pepper, julienned 1 1/2 lb. broccoli, sliced into florets Salt and pepper to taste 2 lemons, sliced in half

Direction

Preheat your grill to medium-high. In a bowl, mix 1 tablespoon oil, garlic, broth and chili. Heat in a pan over medium heat for 30 seconds. In another bowl, toss the broccoli florets in salt, pepper and remaining oil. Grill the broccoli florets for 10 minutes. Grill the lemon slices for 5 minutes. Toss the grilled broccoli and lemon in chili garlic oil. Store in a food container and reheat before serving.

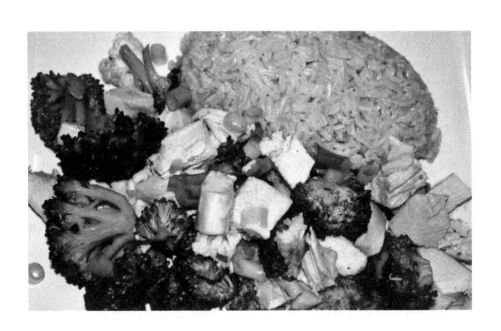

Risotto with Tomato & Herbs

Preparation Time: 10 minutes Cooking Time: 20 minutes

Servings: 32

Ingredients:

2 oz. Arborio rice 1 teaspoon dried garlic, minced 3 tablespoons dried onion, minced 1 tablespoon dried Italian seasoning, crushed ¾ cup snipped dried tomatoes 1 ½ cups reduced-sodium chicken broth

Direction

Make the dry risotto mix by combining all the Ingredients except broth in a large bowl. Divide the mixture into eight resealable plastic bags. Seal the bag. Store at room temperature for up to 3 months. When ready to serve, pour the broth in a pot. Add the contents of 1 plastic bag of dry risotto mix. Bring to a boil and then reduce heat. Cover the pot and simmer for 20 minutes. Serve with vegetables.

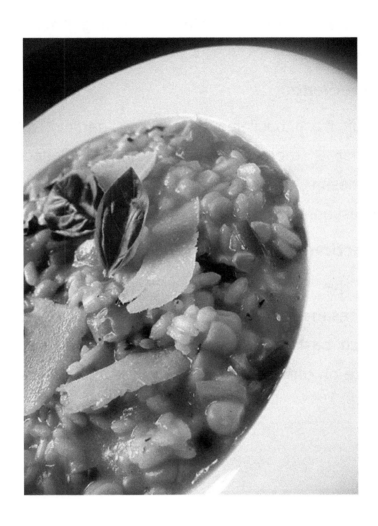

Pesto Pasta

Preparation Time: 10 minutes Cooking Time: 8 minutes
Servings: 2

Ingredients:

1 cup fresh basil leaves 4 cloves garlic 2 tablespoons
walnut 2 tablespoons olive oil 1 tablespoon vegan
Parmesan cheese 2 cups cooked penne pasta 2
tablespoons black olives, sliced

Direction

Put the basil leaves, garlic, walnut, olive oil and
Parmesan cheese in a food processor. Pulse until smooth.
Divide pasta into 2 food containers. Spread the basil
sauce on top. Top with black olives. Store until ready to
serve.

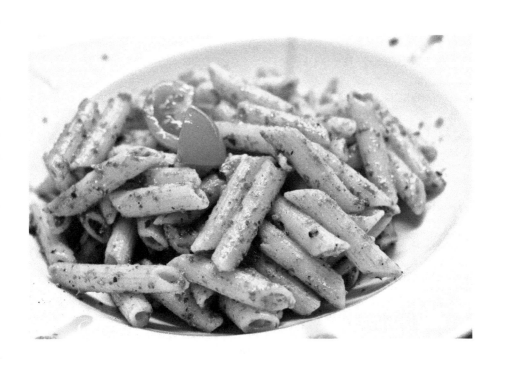

Grilled Summer Veggies

Preparation Time: 15 minutes Cooking Time: 6 minutes

Servings: 6

Ingredients:

2 teaspoons cider vinegar

1 tablespoon olive oil

¼ teaspoon fresh thyme, chopped

1 teaspoon fresh parsley, chopped

¼ teaspoon fresh rosemary, chopped

Salt and pepper to taste

1 onion, sliced into wedges

2 red bell peppers, sliced

3 tomatoes, sliced in half

6 large mushrooms, stems removed

1 eggplant, sliced crosswise

3 tablespoons olive oil

1 tablespoon cider vinegar

Direction Make the dressing by mixing the vinegar, oil, thyme, parsley, rosemary, salt and pepper. In a bowl, mix the onion, red bell pepper, tomatoes, mushrooms and eggplant. Toss in remaining olive oil and cider vinegar. Grill over medium heat for 3 minutes. Turn the vegetables and grill for another 3 minutes. Arrange grilled vegetables in a food container. Drizzle with the herbed mixture when ready to serve.

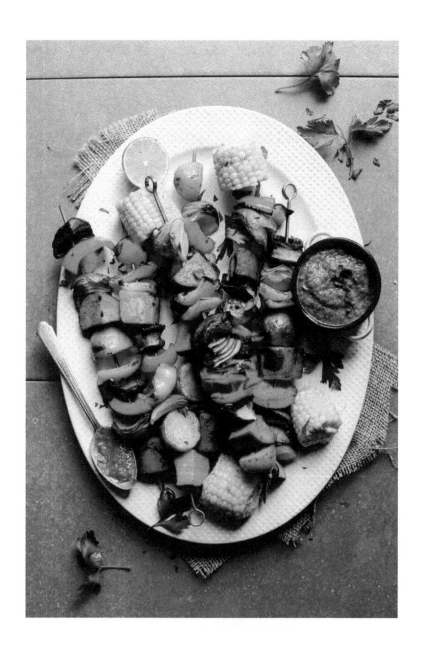

Green Beans with Grape Tomatoes

Preparation time: 10 minutes Cooking time: 20 minutesServings: 8.

Ingredients:

3 pints grape tomatoes 3 tbsp. olive oil salt and pepper to taste 15 ounces green beans

Directions:

Begin by preheating the oven to 350 degrees Fahrenheit. Slice the tomatoes and coat them in olive oil and salt and pepper. Place them in a baking sheet, and cover them with foil. Bake them for sixty minutes. Next, pour oil over the green beans and salt and pepper them. Place them on a baking sheet, and cover them with foil. Broil the beans for six minutes on high, and then toss the greens with the tomatoes. Enjoy.

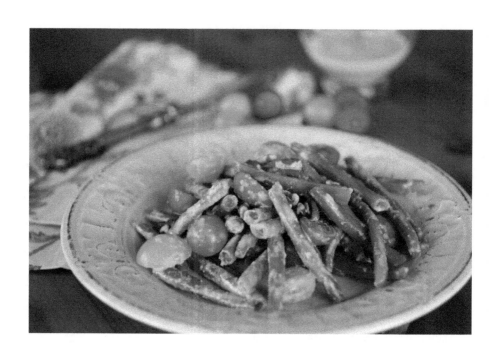

Thanksgiving Cranberry Sauce

Preparation time: 10 minutes Cooking time: 30 minutes Servings: 8.

Ingredients:

16 ounces frozen cranberries 1 cup sugar 1 ½ cup water 1/3 cup tangerine juice zest from 1 tangerine

Directions:

Begin by heating together all of the above ingredients in a saucepan. Stir every few minutes. After fifteen minutes, the sauce will thicken. At this time, take the sauce off the heat, allow it to cool, and then chill it in the refrigerator. Enjoy whenever you please!

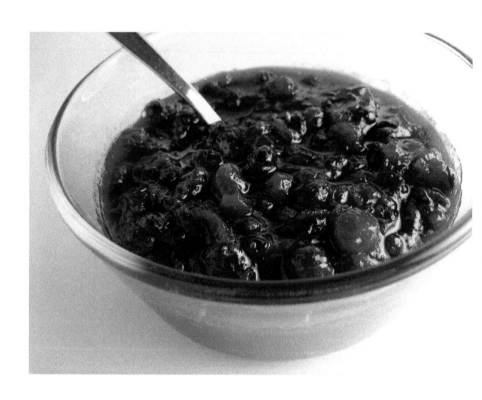

Mapled Carrots with Dill Seasoning

Preparation time: 10 minutes Cooking time: 50 minutesServings: 4.

Ingredients:

2 tbsp. vegan butter 4 cups sliced carrots 2 tbsp. chopped dill 2 tbsp. brown sugar salt and pepper to taste

Directions:

Begin by placing the carrots in a skillet. Add water, and cover the carrots. Allow the mixture to boil. After the water evaporates, add the butter, the dill, the brown sugar, and the salt and pepper. Enjoy warm.

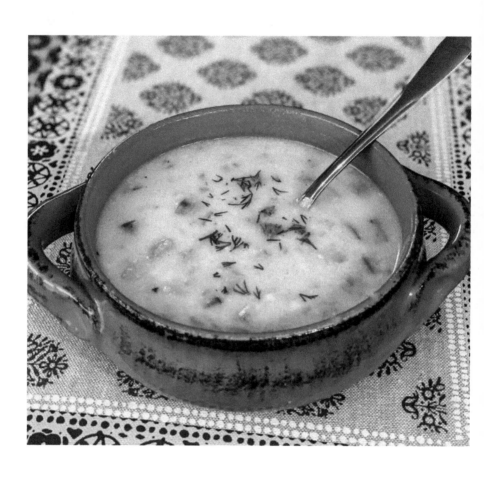

Lemony Snicket Garlic Broccoli

Preparation time: 10 minutes Cooking time: 20 minutesServings: 5.

Ingredients:

2 chopped heads of broccoli 3 tbsp. olive oil 2 minced garlic cloves ½ tsp. lemon juice salt and pepper to taste

Directions:

Begin by preheating the oven to 400 degrees Fahrenheit. Next, toss the broccoli with the salt, pepper, oil, and lemon. Bake the broccoli in the oven for twenty minutes. Add a bit more lemon juice, if you desire, and serve warm.

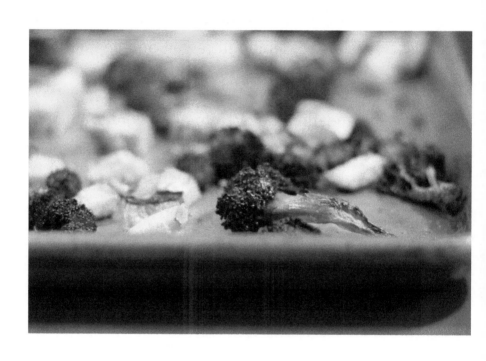

Roasted Cauliflower

Preparation time: 10 minutes Cooking time: 40 minutesServings: 6.

Ingredients:

3 tbsp. minced garlic 1 chopped head of cauliflower 4 tbsp. olive oil salt and pepper to taste

Directions:

Begin by preheating the oven to 450 degrees Fahrenheit. Next, pour the garlic and the olive oil together in a large bag. Add the cauliflower to the bag, and completely coat the cauliflower. Next, pour this mixture into the baking dish, and salt and pepper the creation. Next, bake the mixture for thirty minutes, making sure to stir after fifteen. Add some vegan cheese at the end, if you please, and enjoy.

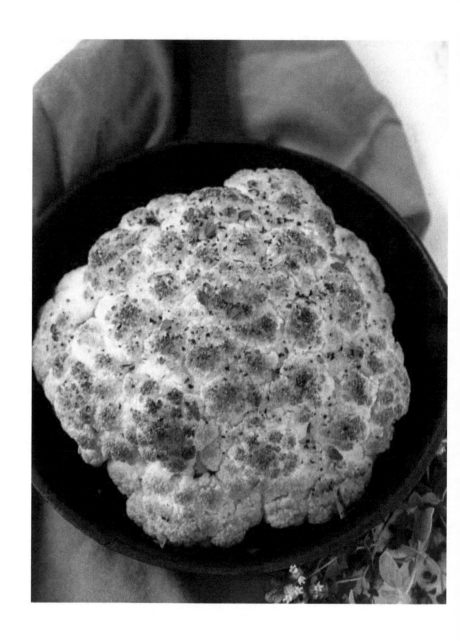

Creamed Fall Corn

Preparation time: 10 minutes Cooking time: 30 minutesServings: 8.

Ingredients:

10 ounces corn 2 tbsp. vegan butter 1 cup vegan cream 2 tbsp. flour 2 tbsp. sugar 1 cup almond milk 1/3 cup chopped vegan Parmesan cheese salt and pepper to taste

Directions:

Begin by heating the cream, the corn, the salt, the sugar, the butte,r and the pepper together in a skillet over medium heat. Continue to stir as you add the milk and the flour. Cook this mixture until the mixture is thick and the corn is cooked. Serve warm with a topping of vegan Parmesan cheese and enjoy.

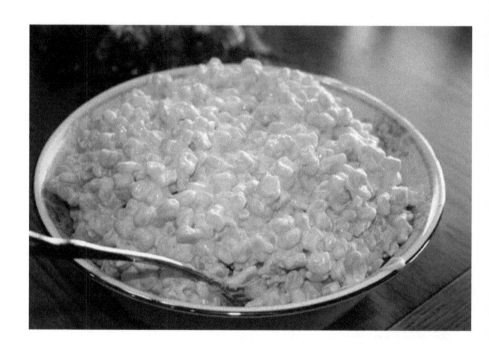

Southern Living Collard Greens

Preparation time: 10 minutes Cooking time: 20 minutesServings: 6.

Ingredients:

1 pound diced collard greens 1 tbsp. olive oil 4 slices cooked tempeh 2 minced garlic cloves 1 diced onion 3 cups vegetable broth salt and pepper to taste

Directions:

Begin by heating the oil and the tempeh together in a big pot over medium heat. After the tempeh becomes crisp, remove the tempeh and crumble it. Return the tempeh to the pan along with the onion, the garlic, and the collard greens. Cook this mixture for five minutes. Next, add the vegetable broth and the salt and pepper. Place the heat on low, and cover the pot. Cook the pot for forty-five minutes, and enjoy!

Super Summer Grilled Zucchini Flats

Preparation time: 10 minutes Cooking time: 30 minutesServings: 4.

Ingredients:

3 length-wise sliced zucchinis 2 tbsp. olive oil

Directions:

Begin by preheating the grill to medium heat. Next, drizzle the oil over the slices of zucchini, and grill the zucchini pieces on the grill for about five minutes per side. Enjoy!

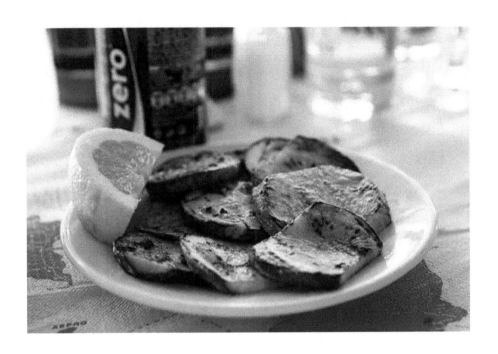

Salty Squash Fries

Preparation time: 10 minutes Cooking time: 30 minutesServings: 4.

Ingredients:

1 halved and de-seeded butternut squash salt to taste

Directions:

Begin by preheating your oven to 425 degrees Fahrenheit. Next, slice the peel from the squash, and slice the squash into fry-like pieces. Arrange these pieces on the baking sheet, and bake the fries for twenty minutes, making sure to spin them over once or twice. After the fries become crispy, pull them out, allow them to cool for a moment, and enjoy!

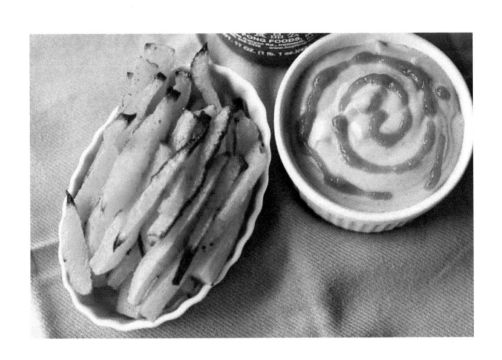

Glazed-Over Mustard Greens

Preparation time: 10 minutes Cooking time: 20 minutesServings: 4.

Ingredients:

1 tsp sesame oil

1 tbsp. sesame seeds

2 tbsp. soy sauce

1 tsp. sake

3 tsp. rice wine

1/3 cup water

7 cups mustard greens

2 tsp. minced garlic

Directions:

Begin by placing the seeds in a skillet over medium. Cook them until they're toasted. Next, add the seeds to a side bowl. Add the sesame oil to the skillet and heat this for two minutes. Add the greens, next, and the water. Stir the greens for two minutes before adding the soy sauce, the garlic, the vinegar, and the sake. Next, allow the mixture to boil. Cover the skillet and allow it to simmer for fifteen minutes. Serve the greens with the sesame seeds, and enjoy.

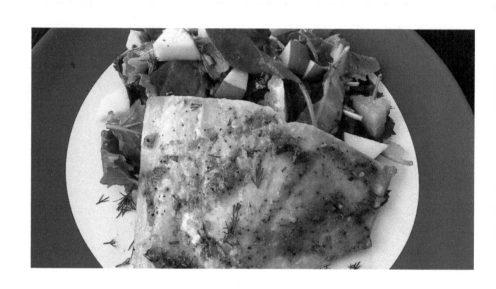

Garlic-Based Spinach Side

Preparation time: 10 minutes Cooking time: 40 minutesServings: 4.

Ingredients:

10 ounces spinach 1 tbsp. vegan butter 7 minced garlic cloves juice from one lemon 1 tsp. garlic salt

Directions:

Begin by melting the vegan butter in a skillet. Add the garlic and stir for two minutes. Next, add the spinach and allow it to wilt for five minutes. Lastly, add the lemon juice and a bit of garlic salt, and serve warm.

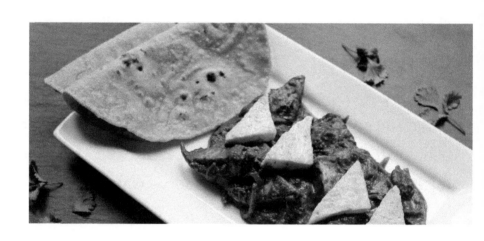

Lemoned Chard

Preparation time: 10 minutes Cooking time: 50 minutesServings: 4.

Ingredients:

4 cups packed rainbow chard 5 tbsp. olive oil 7 minced garlic cloves ½ tsp. reed pepper flakes 1 ½ tbsp. lemon juice

Directions:

Begin by removing the stems from the chard. Heat the olive oil in a skillet along with the garlic, the chard stems, and the red pepper flakes. Cook this mixture for three minutes. Next, add the chard leaves, and cover the mixture for five minutes. Stir and add the lemon juice. After three more minutes of stirring and cooking, serve the chard warm. Enjoy. Fall Time Side:

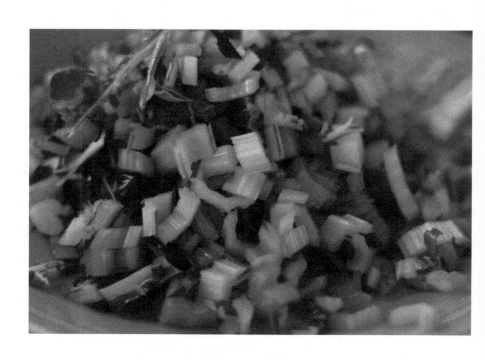

Apples and Sweet Potatoes

Preparation time: 10 minutes Cooking time: 50 minutesServings: 6.

Ingredients:

2 diced and peeled sweet potatoes 1 tsp. allspice 3 tbsp. vegan butter 1/3 cup white sugar 1 peeled and sliced apple ¼ cup soymilk 1 tsp. cinnamon

Directions:

Begin by bringing the sweet potato chunks together in a saucepan with water. Allow the water to boil for twenty minutes. Next, melt the vegan butter in a skillet along with the spices and the sugar. Add the sliced apples to this mixture, and simmer the mixture, covered, for seven minutes. Next, mix the apples with the cooked sweet potatoes—out of the water—and add the soymilk. Mix well with a fork or a mixer, and mash the potatoes well. Enjoy warm.

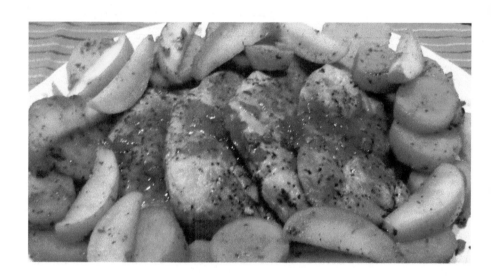

Leeks Medley

Preparation Time: 10 minutes Cooking Time: 12 minutes

Servings:

Ingredients

6 leeks, roughly chopped 1 tablespoon cumin, ground 1 tablespoon mint, chopped 1 tablespoon parsley, chopped 1 teaspoon garlic, minced A drizzle of olive oil Salt and black pepper to the taste

Directions:

In a pan that fits your Air Fryer, combine leeks with cumin, mint, parsley, garlic, salt, pepper and the oil, toss, introduce in your Air Fryer and cook at 350 ° F for 12 minutes. Divide leeks medley between plates and serve as a side dish.

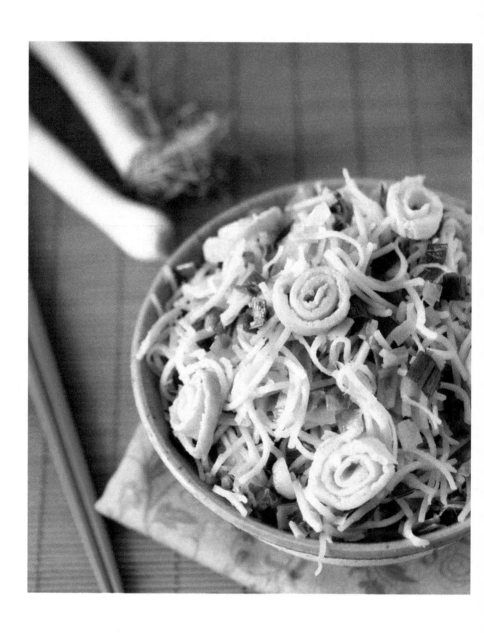

Corn and Tomatoes

Preparation Time: 10 minutes Cooking Time: 13 minutes

Servings:

Ingredients

2 cups corn 4 tomatoes, roughly chopped 1 tablespoon olive oil Salt and black pepper to the taste 1 tablespoon oregano, chopped 1 tablespoon parsley, chopped 2 tablespoons soft tofu, pressed and crumbled

Directions:

In a pan that fits your Air Fryer, combine corn with tomatoes, oil, salt, pepper, oregano and parsley, toss, introduce the pan in your Air Fryer and cook at 320 ° F for 10 minutes. Add tofu, toss, introduce in the fryer for 3 minutes more, divide between plates and serve as a side dish.

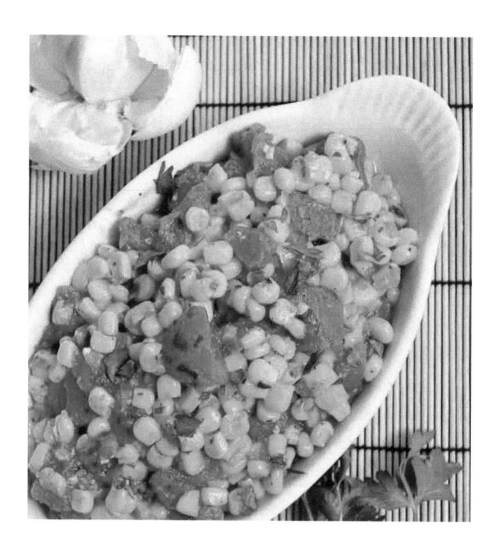

Collard Greens Delight

Preparation Time: 10 minutes Cooking time: 4 hours and 5 minutes Servings: 4

Ingredients:

1 tablespoons olive oil 1 cup yellow onion, chopped 16 ounces collard greens 2 garlic cloves, minced A pinch of sea salt Black pepper to the taste 14 ounces veggie stock 1 bay leaf 1 tablespoon agave nectar 3 tablespoon balsamic vinegar

Directions:

Heat up a pan with the oil over medium high heat, add onion, stir and cook for 3 minutes. Add collard greens, stir, cook for 2 minutes more and transfer to your slow cooker. Add garlic, salt, pepper, stock and bay leaf, stir, cover and cook on Low for 4 hours. In a bowl, mix vinegar with agave nectar and whisk well. Add this to collard greens, stir, divide between plates and serve. Enjoy!

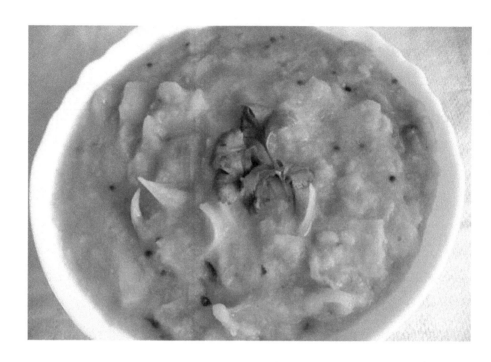

Amazing Carrots Surprise

Preparation Time: 10 minutes Cooking time: 8 hours
Servings: 12

Ingredients:

3 pounds carrots, peeled and cut into medium pieces A
pinch of sea salt Black pepper to the taste 2 tablespoons
water ½ cup agave nectar 2 tablespoons olive oil ½
teaspoon orange rind, grated

Directions:

Put the oil in your slow cooker and add the carrots. In a
bowl mix agave nectar with water and whisk well. Add
this to your slow cooker as well. Also, add a pinch of sea
salt and black pepper, stir gently everything, cover and
cook on Low for 8 hours. Sprinkle orange rind all over,
stir gently, divide on plates and serve. Enjoy!

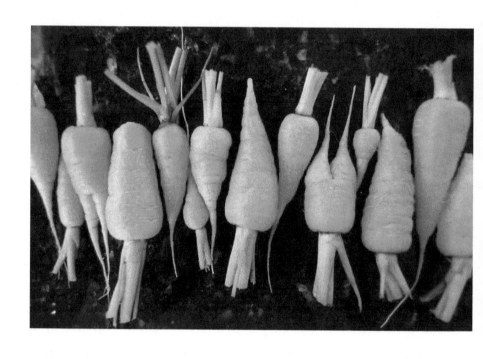

Flavored Beets

Preparation Time: 10 minutes Cooking time: 8 hours Servings: 6

Ingredients:

6 beets, peeled and cut into wedges

A pinch of sea salt Black pepper to the taste

 2 tablespoons lemon juice

2 tablespoons olive oil

2 tablespoons agave nectar

1 tablespoon cider vinegar

½ teaspoon lemon rind, grated

2 rosemary sprigs

Directions:

Put the beets in your slow cooker. Add a pinch of salt, black pepper, lemon juice, oil, agave nectar, rosemary and vinegar. Stir everything, cover and cook on Low for 8 hours. Add lemon rind, stir, divide between plates and serve. Enjoy!

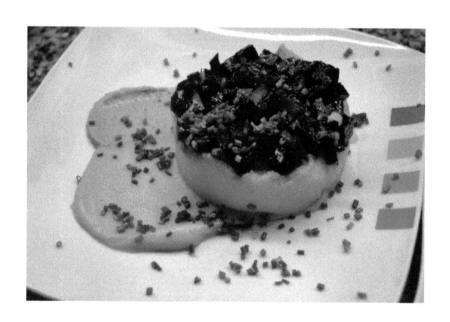

Easy Sweet Potatoes Dish

Time: 30 minutes Cooking time: 2 hours Servings: 6

Ingredients:

4 pounds sweet potatoes, peeled and sliced ½ cup orange juice 3 tablespoons palm sugar Black pepper to the taste ½ teaspoon sage, dried 2 tablespoons olive oil

Directions:

Put the oil in your slow cooker and add sweet potato slices. Add this over potatoes, toss to coat, cover slow cooker and cook on Low for 6 hours. Stir sweet potatoes mix again, divide between plates and serve. Enjoy!

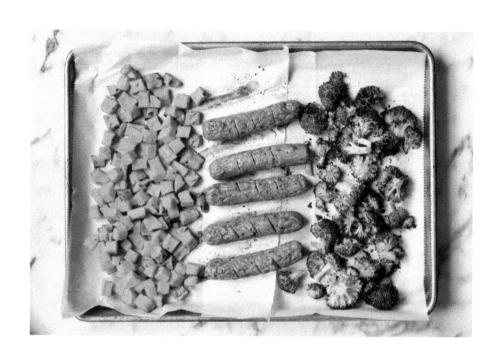

Delicious Mashed Potatoes

Preparation Time: 10 minutes Cooking time: 6 hours Servings: 12

Ingredients:

3 pounds russet potatoes, peeled and cubed

6 garlic cloves, chopped

28 ounces veggie stock

1 bay leaf

1 cup coconut milk

¼ cup coconut butter

A pinch of sea salt

White pepper to the taste

Directions:

Put potatoes in your slow cooker. Add stock, garlic and bay leaf, stir, cover and cook on Low for 6 hours. Drain potatoes, discard bay leaf, return them to your slow cooker and mash using a potato masher. Meanwhile, put the coconut milk in a pot, stir and heat up over medium heat. Add coconut butter and stir until it dissolves. Add this to your mashed potatoes, season with a pinch of salt and white pepper, stir well, divide between plates and serve as a side dish. Enjoy!

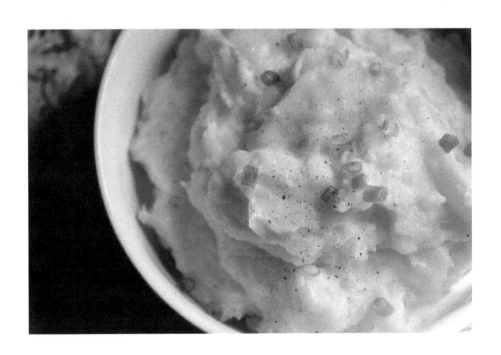

Beans, Carrots and Spinach Side Dish

Preparation Time: 10 minutes Cooking time: 4 hours Servings: 6

Ingredients:

5 carrots, sliced

1 and ½ cups great northern beans, dried, soaked overnight and drained

2 garlic cloves, minced

1 yellow onion, chopped

Salt and black pepper to the taste

½ teaspoon oregano, dried

5 ounces baby spinach

4 and ½ cups veggie stock

2 teaspoons lemon peel, grated

3 tablespoons lemon juice

1 avocado, pitted, peeled and chopped

¾ cup tofu, firm, pressed, drained and crumbled

¼ cup pistachios, chopped

Directions:

In your slow cooker, mix beans with onion, carrots, garlic, salt, pepper, oregano and veggie stock, stir, cover and cook on High for 4 hours. Drain beans mix, return to your slow cooker and reserve ¼ cup cooking liquid. Add spinach, lemon juice and lemon peel, stir and leave aside for 5 minutes. Transfer beans, carrots and spinach mixture to a bowl, add pistachios, avocado, tofu and reserve cooking liquid, toss, divide between plates and serve as a side dish. Enjoy!

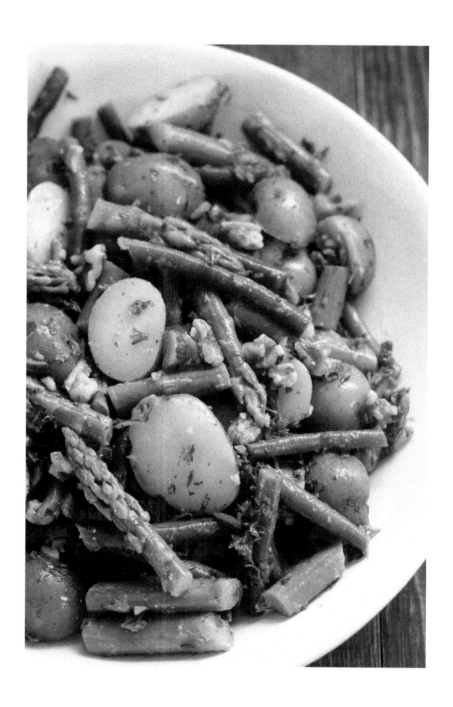

All Beet Up Sweet Potato

Preparation time: 10 minutes Cooking time: 25 minutes Servings: 6.

Ingredients:

7 diced beets 3 tbsp. olive oil 1 tsp. garlic powder 4 diced sweet potatoes 1 diced onion salt and pepper to taste

Directions:

Begin by preheating your oven to 400 degrees Fahrenheit. Next, toss the beets with 1 tbsp. of olive oil, and spread this beet layer in a baking sheet. Add the rest of the olive oil, the salt, the pepper, the garlic powder, the sweet potatoes, and the onions together in a plastic bag, and shake the bag in order to coat the vegetables. Next, bake the beets for fifteen minutes. Add the sweet potatoes, next, and allow the mixture to bake for an additional fifty minutes. Make sure to stir every twenty minutes or so. Serve the mixture warm, and enjoy!

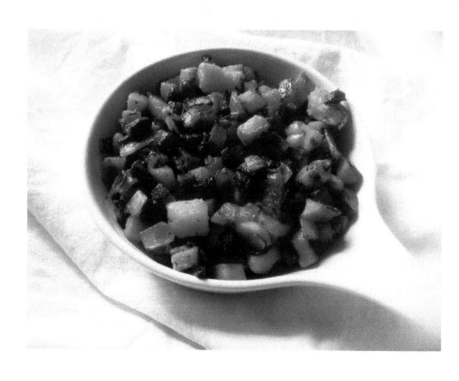

Currant is Current Applesauce

Preparation time: 10 minutes Cooking time: 35 minutesServings: 8.

Ingredients:

12 peeled and sliced apples 6 peeled and sliced peaches ½ cup herbal tea 1 tsp. ginger 4 cups red currants 1 tbsp. marjoram ½ tsp. allspice

Directions:

Begin by forming all the above ingredients except for the currants together in a large soup pot. Place the heat to medium-high, and cook and stir the mixture for thirty minutes. Next, remove all excess liquid. Add the currants, and stir well before serving warm or cold.

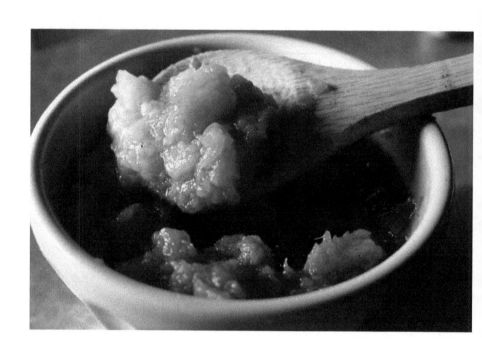

Craving Craisin Bulguar

Preparation time: 10 minutes Cooking time: 25 minutesServings: 2.

Ingredients:

1 tbsp. vegan butter ½ cup dry bulgur wheat 1/3 cup craisins 1/2 cup water 2 tbsp. vegetable stock

Directions:

Begin by allowing the water to boil in a bot. Add the vegetable stock, the vegan butter, and the bulgur to the mix. Cover this mix, and allow the bulgur to simmer for twenty minutes. Next, fluff this mixture and add the craisins. Season as you like, and enjoy warm.

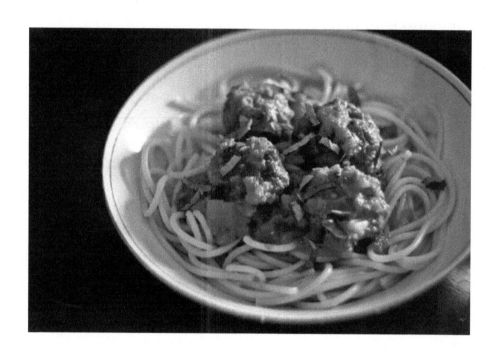

Garbanzo-Based Quinoa

Preparation time: 10 minutes Cooking time: 20 minutesServings: 3 cups.

Ingredients:

2 cups water 1 ¼ cup quinoa ¼ tsp. salt 1 diced tomato 1 cup garbanzo beans 1 tsp. cumin 5 tsp. olive oil 4 tbsp. lime juice 2 minced garlic cloves salt and pepper to taste

Directions:

Begin by bringing the quinoa and a bit of salt into a saucepan of water and allowing it to simmer, covered, for thirty minutes. Next, add the tomatoes, the garbanzo beans, the garlic, the lime juice, and the olive oil to the mix. Add all the spices, and serve warm. Enjoy.

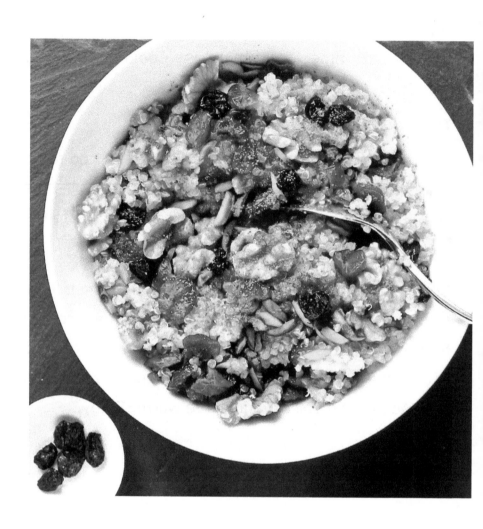

Garlic Mashed Potatoes

Preparation time: 10 minutes Cooking time: 40 minutesServings: 4.

Ingredients:

10 cubed red potatoes 3 tsp. minced garlic 3 tbsp. white sugar ½ cup vegan butter 1/3 tsp. garlic powder ½ cup almond milk

Directions:

Begin by placing the potatoes in a soup pot and covering the potatoes with water. Administer one tsp. of garlic to the water and allow the potatoes to boil for fifteen minutes. Next, drain the water from the potatoes, add the vegan butter, and mash the mixture. Add the almond milk, the sugar, the garlic powder, and all the other garlic. Continue to mix the potatoes until you've created mashed potatoes, and enjoy.

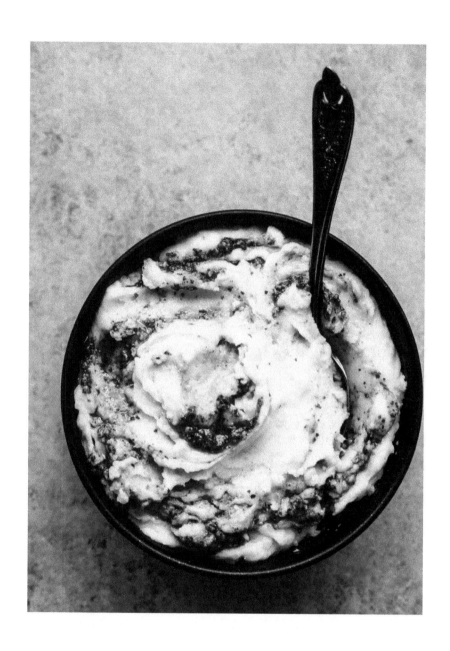

Sweet Mashed Carrots and Potatoes

Preparation time: 10 minutes Cooking time: 45 minutesServings: 6.

Ingredients:

15 ounces baby carrots 1 cubed sweet potato 1/3 cup applesauce 1/3 cup vegan butter 1/3 cup brown sugar 1/3 cup raisins

Directions:

Begin by pouring the potatoes and the carrots together in a soup pot. Cover the vegetables with water, and allow the mixture to simmer for thirty minutes. Drain the mixture of water. Next, melt the vegan butter in a saucepan, and add the brown sugar and the applesauce. Stir well. Afterwards, mash the potatoes and carrots together with the applesauce mixture and the raisins. Enjoy warm.

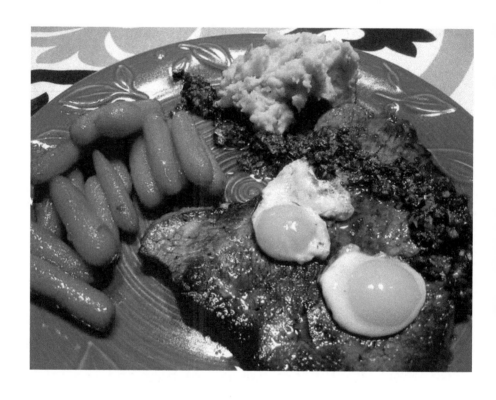

Easy Microwavable Baked Potato

Preparation time: 10 minutes Cooking time: 20 minutesServings: 1 potato.

Ingredients:

1 potato 1 tbsp. vegan butter 3 tbsp. vegan cheddar cheese 4 tsp. vegan sour cream salt and pepper to taste

Directions:

Begin by place the potato on a microwave-safe place, and pricking it with your fork. Cook the potato for five minutes on high. Turn the potato upside down, and cook the potato for an additional five minutes. Afterwards, slice the potato in the center, and add the butter, the salt, the pepper, and a bit of the cheese. Allow the potato to cook for one more minute to melt the cheese, and then add the sour cream. Enjoy.

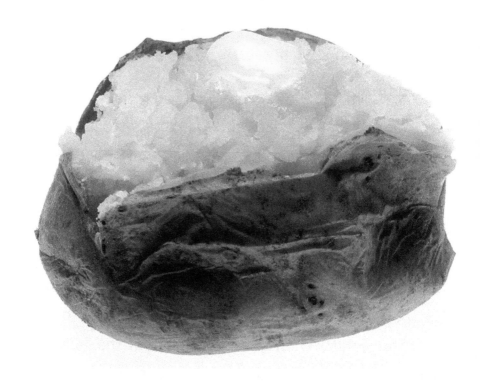

Broccoli and Rice Evening Casserole

Preparation time: 10 minutes Cooking time: 20 minutesServings: 10.

Ingredients:

16 ounces cubed vegan cheddar cheese

20 ounces frozen broccoli

4 cups instant rice

20 ounces coconut milk—without the water (just the cream)

1 cup water

1 diced celery

1 diced onion salt and pepper to taste

Directions:

Begin by cooking both the broccoli and rice together in a saucepan, simmering the water for around twenty minutes. Preheat your oven to 350 degrees Fahrenheit. Next, mix together the cream of the coconut milk and the water. Add the cheese to the saucepan, and mix the ingredients together slowly over medium heat, allowing the cheese to melt. The cheese shouldn't burn. Next, add the vegan butter to a skillet, and add the onion and the celery to the skillet, stirring all the time. To the side in a mixing bowl, place the rice, the broccoli, the cheese mix, the onion, and the celery. Season this mixture with pepper and salt, and add the mixture to a 9x13 pan. Allow the mixture to bake for fifty minutes. It should be golden-brown. Serve warm, and enjoy!

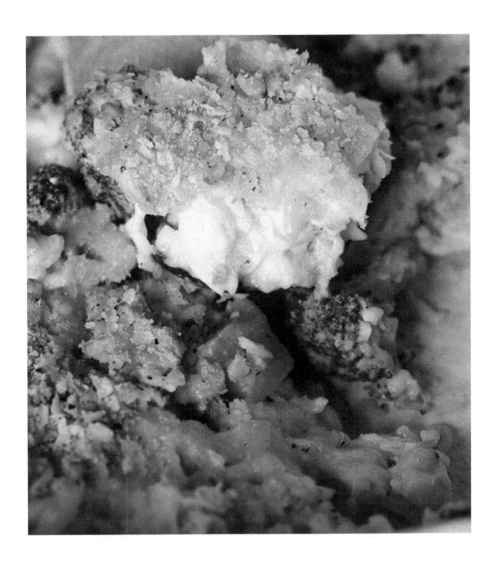

Coconut Cauliflower Rice

Preparation time: 5 minutes Cooking time: 15 minutes Servings: 3

Ingredients:

1 head cauliflower, grated ½ cup heavy cream ¼ cup butter, melted 3 cloves of garlic, minced 1 onion, chopped What you'll need from the store cupboard: Salt and pepper to taste

Directions

Place a nonstick saucepan on high fire and heat cream and butter. Saute onion and garlic for 3 minutes. Stir in grated cauliflower. Season with pepper and salt. Cook until cauliflower is tender, around 5 minutes. Turn off fire and let it set for 5 minutes. Serve and enjoy.

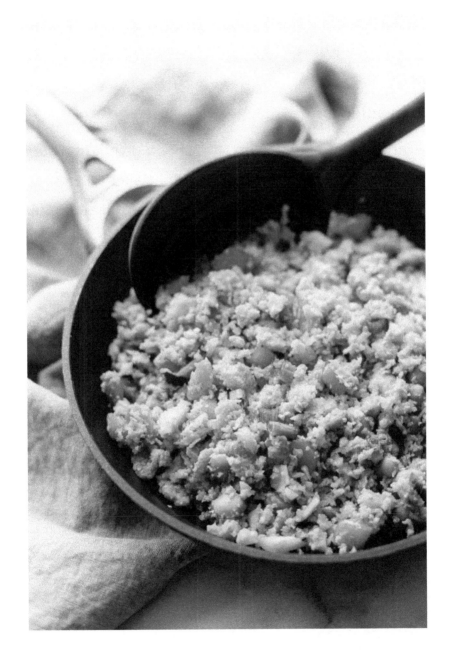

Grilled Cauliflower

Preparation time: 10 minutes Cooking time: 20 minutes Servings: 8

Ingredients:

1 large head cauliflower 1 teaspoon ground turmeric 1/2 teaspoon crushed red pepper flakes Lemon juice, additional olive oil, and pomegranate seeds, optional What you'll need from the store cupboard: 2 tablespoons olive oil 2 tablespoons melted butter

Directions Remove leaves and trim stem from cauliflower. Cut cauliflower into eight wedges. Mix turmeric and pepper flakes. Brush wedges with oil; sprinkle with turmeric mixture. Grill, covered, over medium-high heat or broil 4 minutes from heat until cauliflower is tender, 8-10 minutes on each side. If desired, drizzle with lemon juice and additional oil. Brush with melted butter and serve with pomegranate seeds.

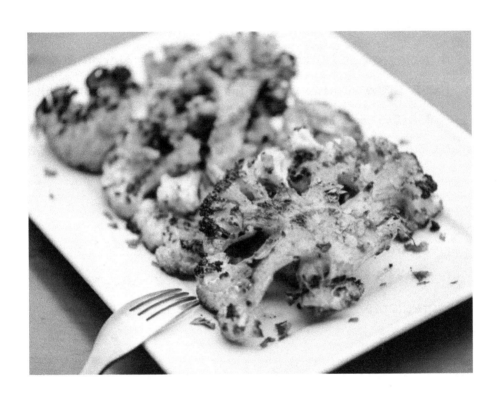

Stir-Fried Buttery Mushrooms

Preparation time: 15 minutes Cooking time: 15 minutes Servings: 4

Ingredients:

4 tablespoons butter 3 cloves of garlic, minced 6 ounces fresh brown mushrooms, sliced 7 ounces fresh shiitake mushrooms, sliced A dash of thyme What you'll need from the store cupboard: 2 tablespoons olive oil Salt and pepper to taste

Directions

Heat the butter and oil in a pot. Sauté the garlic until fragrant, around 2 minutes. Stir in the rest of the ingredients and cook until soft, around 13 minutes.

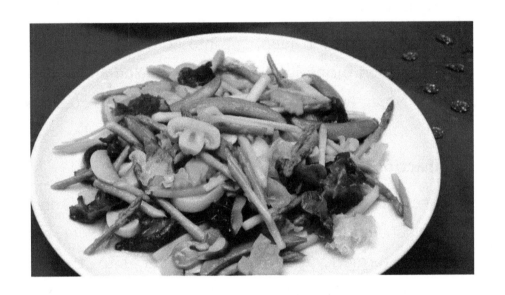

Cauliflower Fritters

Preparation time: 20 minutes Cooking time: 15 minutes Servings: 6

Ingredients:

1 large cauliflower head, cut into florets 2 eggs, beaten ½ teaspoon turmeric 1 large onion, peeled and chopped What you'll need from the store cupboard: ½ teaspoon salt ¼ teaspoon black pepper 6 tablespoons oil

Directions

Place the cauliflower florets in a pot with water. Bring to a boil and drain once cooked. Place the cauliflower, eggs, onion, turmeric, salt, and pepper into the food processor. Pulse until the mixture becomes coarse. Transfer into a bowl. Using your hands, form six small flattened balls and place in the fridge for at least 1 hour until the mixture hardens. Heat the oil in a skillet and fry the cauliflower patties for 3 minutes on each side. Serve and enjoy.

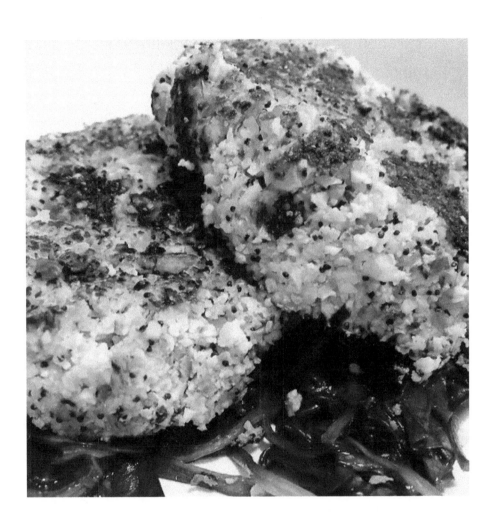

Endives Mix with Lemon Dressing

Preparation time: 15 minutes Cooking time: 0 minutes Servings: 8

Ingredients:

1 bunch watercress (4 ounces) 2 heads endive, halved lengthwise and thinly sliced 1 cup pomegranate seeds (about 1 pomegranate) 1 shallot, thinly sliced 2 lemons, juiced and zested What you'll need from the store cupboard: 1/4 teaspoon salt 1/8 teaspoon pepper 1/4 cup olive oil

Directions

n a large bowl, combine watercress, endive, pomegranate seeds, and shallot. In a small bowl, whisk the lemon juice, zest, salt, pepper, and olive oil. Drizzle over salad; toss to coat.

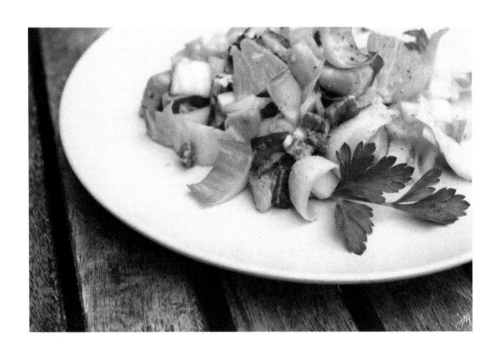

Creamy Artichoke and Spinach

Preparation time: 5 minutes Cooking time: 0 minutes
Servings: 4

Ingredients:

5 tablespoons olive oil

1 can (8 ounces) water-packed artichoke hearts quartered

1 package (3 ounces) frozen spinach

1 cup shredded part-skim mozzarella cheese, divided

1/4 cup grated Parmesan cheese

What you'll need from the store cupboard:

1/2 teaspoon salt 1/4 teaspoon pepper

Directions

Heat oil in a pan over medium flame. Add artichoke hearts and season with salt and pepper to taste. Cook for 5 minutes. Stir in the spinach until wilted. Place in a bowl and stir in mozzarella cheese, Parmesan cheese, salt, and pepper. Toss to combine. Transfer to a greased 2-qt. Broiler-safe baking dish; sprinkle with remaining mozzarella cheese. Broil 4-6 in. from heat 2-3 minutes or until cheese is melted.

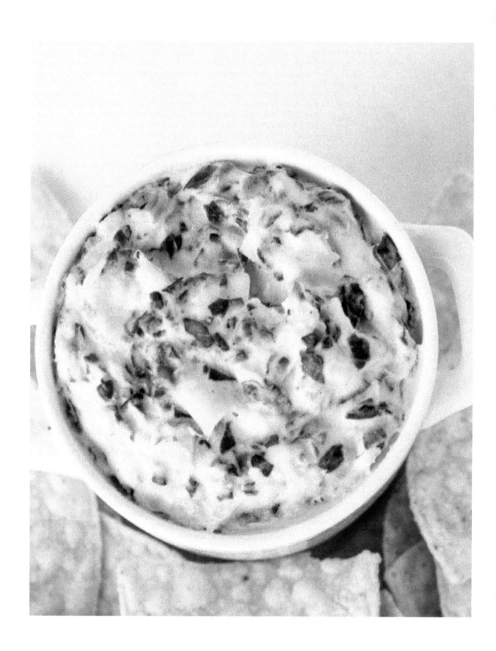

Burrito & Cauliflower Rice Bowl

Preparation Time: 15 minutes Cooking Time: 10 minutes Servings: 4

Ingredients:

1 cup cooked tofu cubes 12 oz. frozen cauliflower rice 4 teaspoons olive oil 1 teaspoon unsalted taco seasoning 1 cup red cabbage, sliced thinly ½ cup salsa ¼ cup fresh cilantro, chopped 1 cup avocado, diced

Direction

Prepare cauliflower rice according to directions in the package. Toss cauliflower rice in olive oil and taco seasoning. Divide among 4 food containers with lid. Top with tofu, cabbage, salsa and cilantro. Seal the container and chill in the refrigerator until ready to serve. Before serving, add avocado slices.

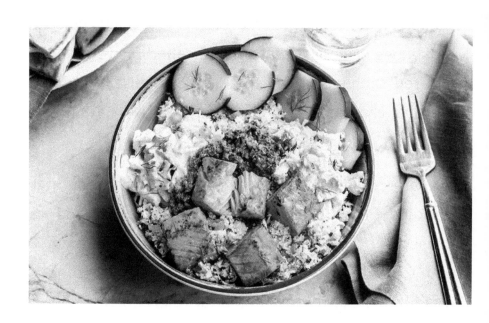

Steamed Cabbage & Carrots

Preparation Time: 10 minutes Cooking Time: 20 minutes Servings: 8

Ingredients:

2 teaspoons olive oil 1 cup carrots, sliced 1 green bell pepper, sliced into strips 1 head green cabbage, sliced 2 tablespoons water Salt and pepper to taste

Direction

Pour oil in a pot over medium heat. Add carrot strips and cook for 5 minutes. Add bell pepper and cabbage. Pour in the water and season with salt and pepper. Cover the pot. Cook for 15 minutes or until tender. Store in food container and reheat when ready to eat.

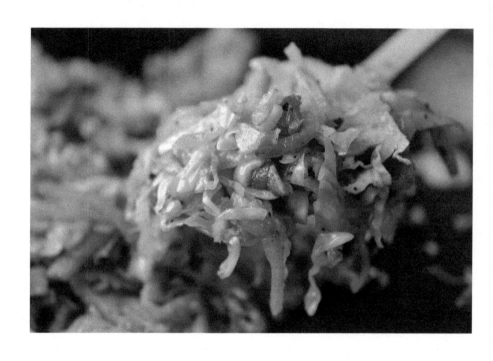

Garlic Pea Shoots

Preparation Time: 5 minutes Cooking Time: 5 minutes Servings: 6

Ingredients:

2 tablespoons canola oil 2 tablespoons sesame oil 3 tablespoons garlic, minced 1 lb. pea shoots ¼ cup rice wine Salt and pepper to taste

Direction

Heat both of the oils in a pot over medium high heat. Add garlic and cook for 30 seconds, stirring frequently. Add pea shoots and rice wine. Season with salt and pepper. Cook for 3 minutes. Place in a food container and heat in the microwave when ready to eat.

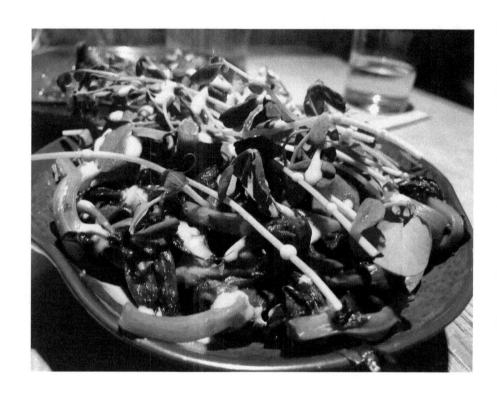

Rustic Mashed Potatoes

Preparation Time: 10 minutes Cooking time: 4 hours Servings: 6

Ingredients:

6 garlic cloves, peeled 3 pounds gold potatoes, peeled and cubed 1 bay leaf 1 cup coconut milk 28 ounces veggie stock 3 tablespoons olive oil Salt and black pepper to the taste

Directions:

In your slow cooker, mix potatoes with stock, bay leaf, garlic, salt and pepper, cover and cook on High for 4 hours. Drain potatoes and garlic, return them to your slow cooker and mash using a potato masher. Add oil and coconut milk, whisk well, divide between plates and serve as a side dish. Enjoy!

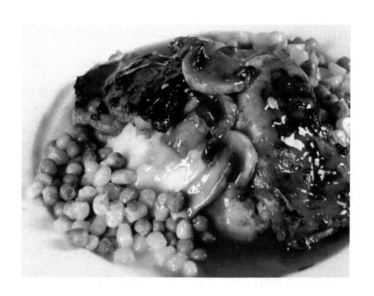

Mushroom and Peas Risotto

Preparation Time: 10 minutes Cooking time: 1 hour and 30 minutes Servings: 8

Ingredients:

1 shallot, chopped 8 ounces white mushrooms, sliced 3 tablespoons olive oil 1 teaspoon garlic, minced 1 and ¾ cup white rice 4 cups veggie stock 1 cup peas Salt and black pepper to the taste

Directions:

In your slow cooker, mix oil with shallot, mushrooms, garlic, rice, stock, peas, salt and pepper, stir, cover and cook on High for 1 hour and 30 minutes. Stir risotto one more time, divide between plates and serve as a side dish. Enjoy!

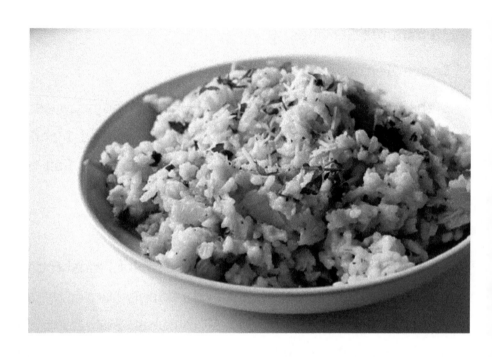

Sizzling Vegetarian Fajitas

Servings: 8 Preparation time: 60 Minutes

Ingredients:

4 ounces of diced green chilies 3 medium-sized tomatoes, diced 1 large green bell pepper, cored and sliced 1 large red bell pepper, cored and sliced 1 medium-sized white onion, peeled and sliced 1/2 teaspoon of garlic powder 1/4 teaspoon of salt 2 teaspoons of red chili powder 2 teaspoons of ground cumin 1/2 teaspoon of dried oregano 1 1/2 tablespoon of olive oil

Directions:

Take a 6-quarts slow cooker, grease it with a non-stick cooking spray and add all the ingredients. Stir until it mixes properly and cover the top. Plug in the slow cooker; adjust the cooking time to 2 hours and let it cook on the high heat setting or until cooks thoroughly. Serve with tortillas.

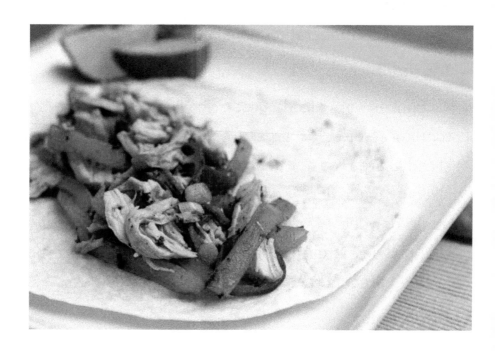